You Can Do This

A Practical Guide to Achieving and Maintaining Your Ideal Weight

by LeeAnne Whitney

I finally did it! So did my husband and you can too. This is a book about our journey. In it we share the things that we learned and implemented in order to reach our goals with the hope that it will help you.

We have kept it very simple on purpose. We choose not to be overly involved in every little detail of the nutritional aspects of the human body. We just want to be healthy & maintain a healthy weight. We keep in mind some basics and go from there while we enjoy life to the fullest.

You can use the knowledge that we have gained and succeed. You'll be in charge of customizing your intake according to your tastes. We hope that you'll enjoy the journey as much as we have. After all that's what inspired the book.

It feels so good to be eating to live instead of living to eat. Join us and experience the joy of a healthy and fulfilling lifestyle.

Ecclesiastes 2:24 There is nothing better for a man, than that he should eat and drink, and that he should make his soul enjoy good in his labor. This also I saw, that it was from the hand of God.

I love to eat! I always have. It's no wonder that I've struggled with weight management most of my life. All I can say is that something finally clicked. I realized that if I was ever going to get it right, it better be now. I'm getting up there. I was inspired by a Pediatrician who was lecturing about the newborn digestive system. He made so much sense. It was all about feeding the body the nutrients it needs and not bogging it down with things that it doesn't need. Wow! How simple is that. As I thought about all of the information that I received in that seminar I developed a plan. I recalled a friend of mine telling me years ago about the system that she used to lose a lot of weight. Many of you are familiar with it. It allots the person cards in several food categories every morning. The person then spends the cards throughout the day and when the cards are gone you stop eating. Voila! My plan was born. I decided to count calories. After about 2 weeks of hearing me say, "guess how many calories are in that?" My husband decided to join me. He's so glad that he did. Hope you decide to join in the fun as well.

I still love eating! Even more than ever because now I have the satisfaction of knowing that I'm fueling my body instead of overtaxing it. Now I decide what to eat based on very basic guidelines as well as appeal. This means a wide variety of delicious and nutritious foods everyday. Yum! Of course we all have our weaknesses and we do indulge on occasion but now we make an educated decision to do so.

The real inspiration for this book was the amount of food that we consume. So many people struggle to limit their intake & we don't have to do that at all. I've said to my husband so many times, "if people could see how much we eat, they'd never believe it." So I decided to show you.

Let's get right to the nitty gritty!

The first thing I did was to determine our daily calorie goals. Easy to do. I went on line and found many sites where I could obtain the information. You can use the sites to track everything. I've included a chart that will help for those of you who don't use the internet. I chose to use good old pencil and paper. I purchased a small notebook and some tabs. I divided it into my section and my husband's. I wrote down our calorie and our weight goals. I designated a few pages to track our daily calorie consumption and weights.

Of course now I needed a calorie counting book. Again the information is available on line but I wanted a mid sized paperback. I ordered it online. Then I began writing down everything that we consumed each day with it's calorie count and with the total at the bottom of the day's page. I also began counting how many foods had protein, fats, or carbs in order to see that our regimen consisted of about 45% carbs *(vegetables, fruits, & whole grains)*, 30% protein *(lean meats, dairy, nuts, etc)* , & 25% healthy fats *(dairy, olive oil, fish oil, etc.)* I'm not an expert on these kind of details. We are healthy eaters and did very well when I tracked this. Our problem was not variety it was calories because we enjoy large portions.

Daily Calorie Intake Guide:

If you weigh <200 lbs. then eat about 1200-1500 calories per day

If your Weight is:	Your Calorie Intake:
200-225 lbs.	1500-1800 daily
226-300 lbs.	1800-2500 daily
301-350 lbs.	2500-3000 daily

Example Entries:

LeeAnne's Progress

Date	Calories	Weight
5/1/13	1205	120
5/2	1193	
5/3	1220	
5/4	1195	119.5
5/5	1300	
5/6	1200	
5/7	1186	119
& so on.		

I went from 140# to 115# in about 6 months. My husband lost 40# during the same time. My calorie goal was 1200 calories while his was 2361. He could just about double my consumption. It was very encouraging to know that the scale had no choice but to go down as we stuck to our plan. I liked writing down the reductions when they occurred. My husband chose to write down daily weights. I have remained steady for 5 months now & stopped counting diligently soon after I reached my goal. Now I watch the scale & adjust accordingly.

Saturday

Coffee	30	
Cereal & Milk	190	
Bran, Raisins, Coconut	90	
Bkft. Total		310
Sandwich	160	
Melon, Yogurt, Honey	137	
Orange	40	
Lunch		337
Steak	250	
Salad	200	
Cucumbers	45	
Brussel Sprouts	50	
Dinner		545
Ice Cream Float	150	
Total		1342

Carbs IIIIIIIIIII   Protein IIIIIII   Fats IIII

Education on the calorie content of everything I put in my mouth was next. I was amazed and you will be, too. I started omitting the higher calorie foods and adding lower calorie choices to our meals and snacks. Shopping was now an adventure and challenge. I love a challenge! Maybe that's why I've enjoyed this so much.

I developed some new lingo through this whole process. I will be using it throughout this book so I want you to understand what I'm saying. I pretended that my 1200 calories was actually $1200. So each morning I got $1200 to spend. Woohoo! I read somewhere that I shouldn't eat less than 1200 calories in a day so I really had to spend it. No savings account. Each day is new and at the end of the day the money is gone. My husband and I began saying things like, " is it affordable? Is it a good deal? Or does it fit into the budget?" Meaning how many calories are in it.

Because I enjoy eating so much, I choose to eat larger portions of low calorie foods instead of smaller portions of higher calorie foods. I think that's a key. We never suffer hunger involuntarily and never feel deprived. I make many substitutions and create many new dishes using lower calorie ingredients. The possibilities are endless. I do not however sacrifice quality. We include a few things because of the health benefits and/or flavor.

Several of these include:

Organic Milk   *Ever done a taste test? Check it out.*
You won't go back.
Raw Local Honey   *Included in our daily regimen due to*
its health benefits.
Raisins   *Reconstituted or dry they are a*
delicious little addition to cereal.
Nut Topping   *I sprinkle chopped nuts on for the*
protein and for the taste.
Fat Free Whipped Cream   *In the can. A staple for me @ 5*
calories for 2 Tablespoons.
Sea Salt or the equivalent   *Has 97 trace minerals in it!*

Use your imagination and adjust according to your tastes!

Staples for us include:

Fresh Fruits
Fresh Vegetables
Lean Meats and Fish
Splenda
Honey
Molly McButter *(in the spice section)*
Low fat Mayonnaise: (*15 calories for 1 Tablespoon instead of 100!*)
Cooking Spray Oils *(0 calories)*
Low Calorie Salad Dressings
Skim Milk

Low Fat Plain Yogurt
Light Sour Cream
Low Calorie Breads *(35 calories per slice and delicious)*
Fat Free Hot Dogs *(50 calories each)*
Turkey Jerky
Salmon, Tuna, Low Calorie Sardines
Salsa
Skim Milk Cheeses
Light Ice Cream
Ice Cream Cones (*small cake type)*
Fat Free Whipped Cream
Nut Topping *(I get out of control with other forms of nuts)*
Sugar Free Jell-O and Pudding
Flavored Rice Cakes
Potato Straws *(I love chips & this is a grand substitute)*
Peanut Butter *(I choose a high quality one. Compare them.)*

My kitchen has been revamped! Gone are the high calorie alternatives to the above mentioned staples. Most condiments are not an issue. Enjoy spices & condiments pretty much at will.

The kitchen must have basic measuring devices and we soon realized that we needed a small digital scale, too. At first we weighed everything that could be weighed. It was very enlightening! The rule of thumb when the scale isn't available is that a meat portion should be about the size of a deck of cards. Whoa! I used to eat the whole Steak & we'd shared a whole Chicken! This was an adjustment for us. We've grown accustomed to smaller meat portions now. We just fill the gaps with loads of low calorie Vegetables and Fruits with small amounts of delectable goodies thrown into the mix.

For example we'll have a large low calorie Vegetable Salad with ½ sliced Avocado, a few sprinkles of Sunflower and Pumpkin Seeds, and a Tablespoon or two of Crumbly Bleu Cheese on it. All topped with a low calorie Italian, Raspberry Vinaigrette, and/or Creamy Bleu Cheese dressings. The trick is not to combine high calorie foods in the same meal. If you're having Potatoes, cut out the Avocado in the Salad, etc.

Helpful Tips!

While we were losing weight we were pretty strict with ourselves. We pretty much cut out Potatoes, Rice, Pasta, high calorie Breads and Dough, Popcorn, etc. *(I always thought that Popcorn was low in calories. Not so.)* Now that we're maintaining we have more leeway because our calorie consumption goal went up! When we exercise it goes up even more. Now we've added Potatoes back into our diets which we enjoy thoroughly. We did enjoy them on occasion while losing, too. We love Popcorn & fit it in when we have room to do so. We also enjoy Rice and

Pasta very occasionally. There is a Tofu pasta type product that is a very good deal for Pasta lovers. We actually enjoy Spaghetti Squash so much that we haven't gone back to Pasta much. I just created a Spinach and Eggplant Lasagna using the Squash instead of noodles that was excellent and affordable. I also recently realized that I can make Pizza that fits into our budget. The key is not to combine high calorie foods, right? So, the crust is the main source of the calories. Tomato sauce is fine. I sauté a bunch of Vegetables like Green Peppers, Onions, Summer Squash, Eggplant and/or Mushrooms and use them as the bulk of the toppings. Use fat free Mozzarella Cheese and a few Pepperonis or Bacon bits and whatever else you like so long as you don't overdo the high calorie items. It's absolutely satisfying!

Another thing that I've implemented is to cook Chicken Breasts in a sealed foil packet. Add different Spices, Onions, Garlic, etc. The possibilities are endless. I love putting a little Buffalo Chicken sauce in there. I cook them @ 350 degrees for 30-40 minutes depending on the size of the Breast. Slice it and serve it with some of the juice. Delicious and very low cal!

A good idea that helps us is to have low calorie snacks and fillers readily available. My husband loves Cucumbers so I keep a bowl of sliced Cucumbers and Onions in a mixture of Vinegar, Water, salt and pepper, and a little Oil in the fridge. Sliced Tomatoes are good in this mix as well. Other things I prepare are Blue Kraut *(German style Red Cabbage)*, Cole Slaw, and fresh Fruit Salads. Melons are an especially good deal.

My poor body has never enjoyed a healthy eating schedule until now. I use to drink 8-10 cups of decaf with cream & sugar til 11 or 12 and then eat a little lunch. Either that or I'd skip eating or drinking anything else until dinner. I've always enjoyed dinner and usually consumed large portions of high calorie foods from dinnertime to bedtime. My dad was famous for the midnight snack. Not necessarily at midnight mind you but late in the evening nonetheless.

Now I drink 3-4 cups of decaf with organic 2% milk in it in the AM without sweetener, eat a healthy breakfast between 9:30 & 10:30, lunch between noon and 3, dinner at suppertime, and multiple desserts and/or snacks til near bedtime. I'm blessed to be able to sleep well on a full stomach.

I'm told that the best way to eat is to *"graze"* all day. That's what I do now. I can tell you that I feel and look much better.

The Bowels

I want to add information here about this very important subject. How very important it is to keep the bowels moving. I know how to do just that. I am an RN and see the problems that unhealthy bowels can cause just about everyday. This issue is huge. Implement this little regimen & you can be among those of us who enjoy regularity.

The recipe that I use:

3 Cups of Wheat Bran *(from a health food store. Not bran cereal)*
1 Quart of Unsweetened Applesauce
Water
(I add about 1/4 cup of water to the applesauce jar & shake it to get all the goodies)

Mix these together & keep refrigerated. Eat near the same time everyday to regulate bowels.

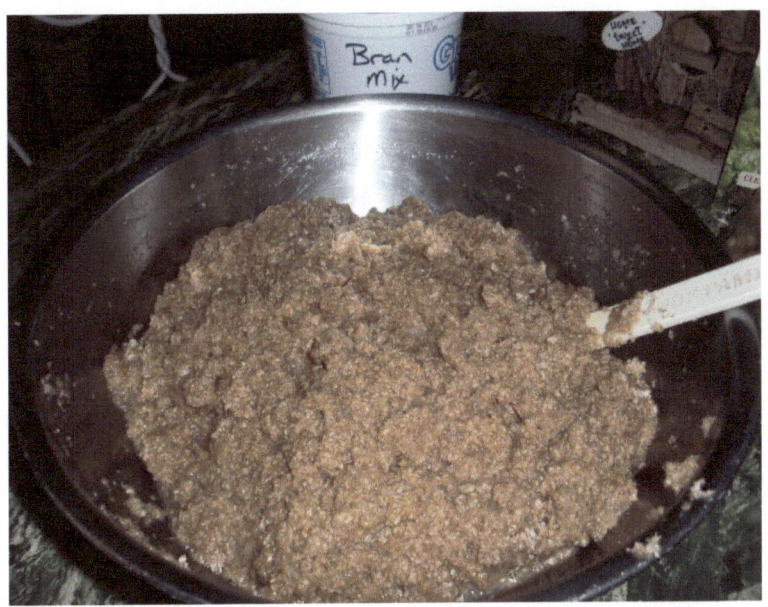

Adjust the amount consumed according to the results.

After some experimentation revealed issues in both directions, I determined that I need to consume about 6 heaping Tablespoons with my breakfast every morning. I may adjust this amount accordingly if I plan to eat foods that tend to constipate or vice versa.

It's good all by itself however I usually start with this mix and then add ¼ cup Yogurt, some fresh Fruit, Raisins, Nut topping, and a Banana. I may add some Honey or Granola bar pieces.

I've seen many constipation issues resolved using a recipe like mine.

The original recipe calls for:

1 cup of Prune Juice, 2 cups of Wheat Bran, and 2 cups of Applesauce.

I modified it to reduce the calorie count.

I calculate about 10 calories per Tablespoon for my mix.

Way back when I was originally inspired, the Pediatrician giving the lecture said that the Banana is one of the most perfect foods. It is easily digested and full of nutrients. I've always loved Bananas but hardly ever enjoyed them. I always felt that they were too fattening. Now I eat one almost everyday.

He also mentioned the benefits of raw local Honey which increases our immunity to local allergens which I try to consume daily as well.

I implement a few good habits like the ones mentioned. I also work to keep a wide variety of selections in our menu. Thank God that I married a man who also loves to eat & will try anything. I serve experiments quite frequently. They are almost always delicious!

Next I'll display a couple of prepared staples in case you'd like to implement them.

Blue Kraut

About 25 Calories per cup

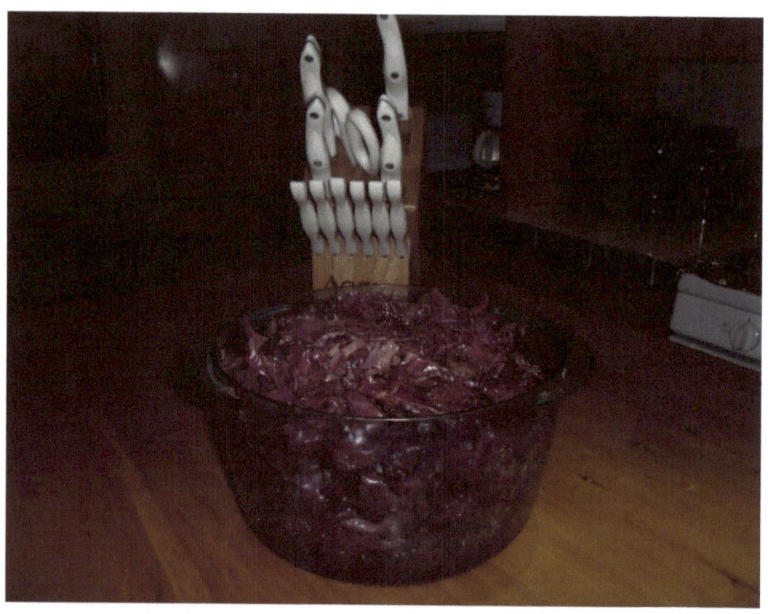

Cut Red Cabbage and put it in a large stockpot. Add 1-2 cut up Apples *(skin, too)*, a cut up Onion or 2, ½ cup of Apple Cider Vinegar, a cup of Water, a Tablespoon or 2 of Apple Pie Spice.

I use Cinnamon, Nutmeg, Cloves, & Allspice. Easy on the Nutmeg and Cloves. I also add some salt or you can wait and salt to taste when done. Simmer this on low heat until soft. It takes an hour or two to cook.

Cucumber Salad
Most of the calories are in the oil.

About 25 calories per cup

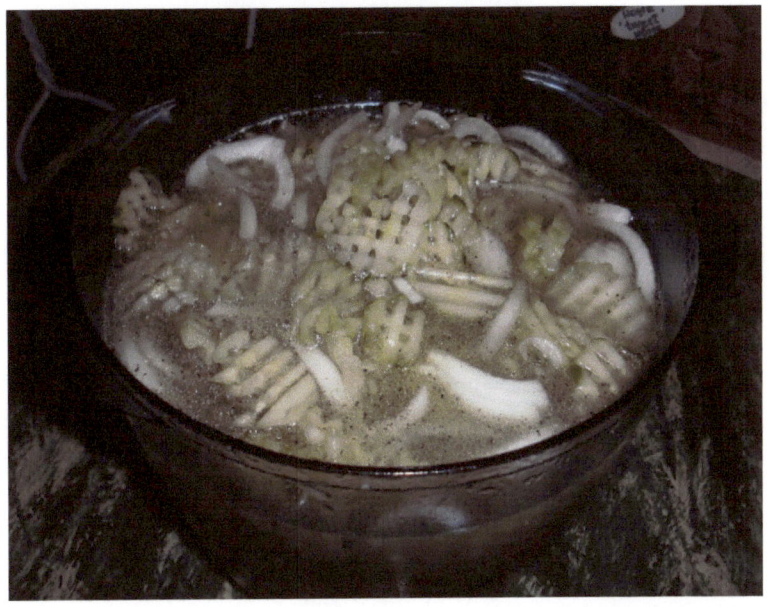

Fill a medium sized bowl 1/2-3/4 full of sliced Cucumbers
with a couple of sliced Onions. Add
Vinegar & a splash of Oil & then add Water enough to
cover the Cucumbers.
We keep the bowl going all season & add splashes of
Vinegar & Oil with each new batch.

More Tips

At each meal eat some protein. It helps you to feel satisfied because your body needs it.

I take a Gummy Multivitamin & sometimes take a Gummy Fish Oil Supplement. They both taste GREAT! I am a healthy eater but felt that this would insure that I am getting everything that my body requires.
Don't forget to count the calories! Worth it in my opinion.

At first I made Herbal Tea with Honey in it & refrigerated it . Then I discovered 0 calorie flavored Waters. I drank a 16 oz. soda just about everyday of my life before this endeavor. 200 calories! Not worth it. There are SO MANY flavors & options for 0 calorie drinks. Check out the drink mixes, additives, & bottled Waters. This one category is a blast because of the variety available. We change it up so as not to get too much of one type of artificial sweetener too often. Moderation in all things is a good motto.

Add exercise to your daily life whenever possible to optimize good health & muscle tone. Exercise will also burn calories and accelerate the weight loss process.
Park near a cart return bin far out instead of close to the entrance when shopping.
Pick up some small dumbbells & begin a short weight lifting routine. *(Caution: don't overdo or lift heavy weights too quickly. That was stupid and it set me back for months.)*

Find an easy routine that includes some exercise moves like squats, leg lifts, etc. & add it to your life a few times a week.
Take a walk, ride a bike, jog, skip rope, hula hoop. Customize at will.

Sometimes we just need to overstuff ourselves. At least I do. Aim for the lowest calorie foods & drinks. Here are the things I go for when I feel like a bottomless pit!

Cucumber dishes, Cabbage dishes, Broccoli, Salads, Sautéed Green Peppers & Onions, Fat Free Hot Dogs wrapped in 35 calorie Bread or Toast. You get the idea!

Ice Cream floats
You can fill up on diet soda & light vanilla ice cream. Just keep pouring the 0 calorie soda in. Try different flavors. My favorite is diet Chocolate Fudge Soda.

Sugar Free Jell-O & fruit
I enjoy Fat Free Whipped Cream on top. Very filling.

Light Ice Cream with whipped Cream, a Cone, & Nut Topping. No deprivation going on here!

Banana Splits are good too if you stay away from high calorie syrups.

Now to show you!

The majority of my book is in picture form for your enjoyment and inspiration. I've included my ideas on food preparation, recipes, & calorie information for you. Hopefully you will find this useful. I've tried to group things together in sensible categories. Take what you like and modify the rest according to your likes and dislikes.

Enjoy!

All calorie counts are approximate of course.

Breakfast:

LW's Breakfast Mix
245 Calories

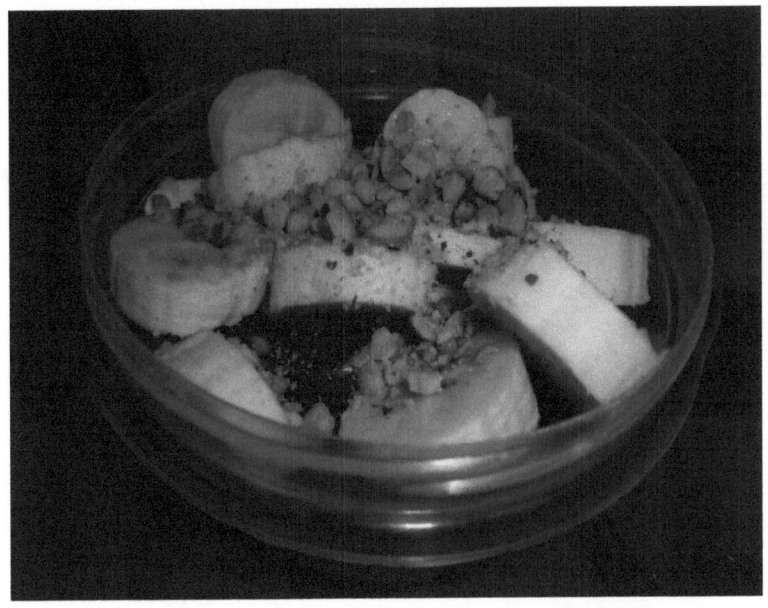

6 T of Bran Mix (60), ¼ c Yogurt (25), Grapes (10) ,1T
Raisins (30), Banana (100), Nuts (20) Coconut is a nice
addition especially with fresh Pineapple or Mango. My
husband usually enjoys a small bowl of Cereal with Organic
Skim Milk, Bran Mix, a Banana, some other Fruit, Yogurt
with more Fruit & Splenda, Tea with honey.

Egg & Cheese English Muffin & Fruit
350 Calories

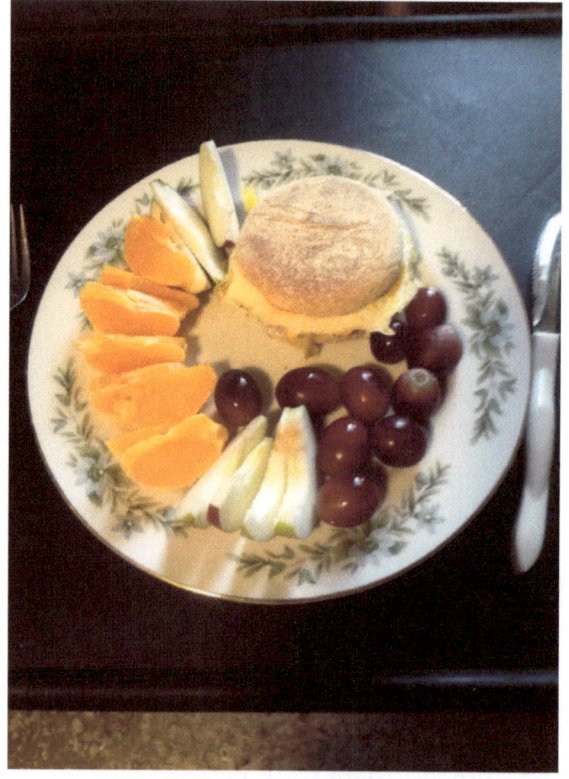

On weekends we sometimes enjoy Eggs, Toast, Hash Brown Potatoes, etc. Just be sure to cook with 0 calorie cooking Oils or perhaps a dash of Olive Oil and use small amounts of Butter or Butter Sprinkles.

A friend of mine uses Egg whites a lot. They are very low calorie & full of protein. I tried making a pancake using them & some fruit but it didn't go well. She does it all the time. Experiment with it!

Lunches:

A typical on the go breakfast & lunch for me.

Lunch 465

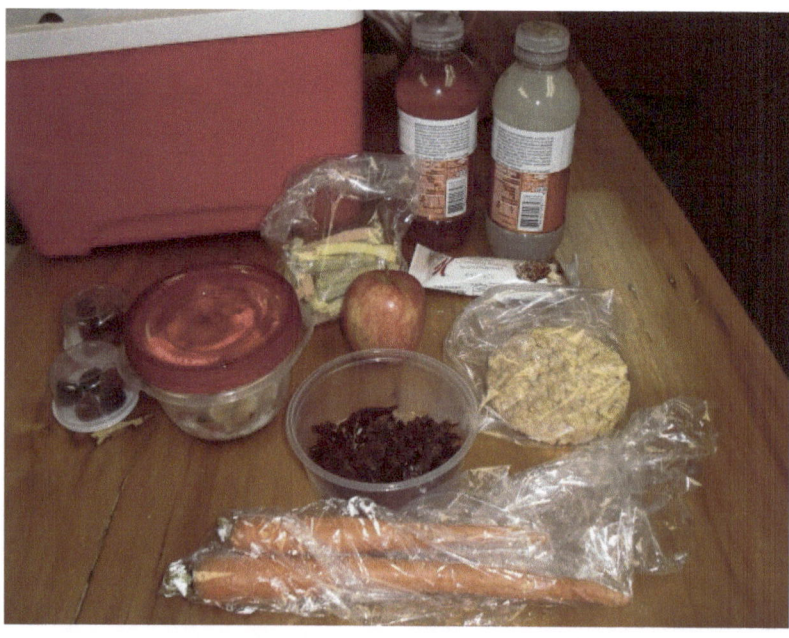

For lunch today: Turkey Jerky (50), Carrots (50), Gummy Vitamins (15), Gummy Fish Oil (35), Potato Straws (100), Apple (70), Caramel Corn Rice Cake (55), Snack Bar (90), 2 flavored Waters(0).

My husband usually enjoys a Sandwich of some type madewith 35 calorie per slice Bread, an Apple, an Orange or other Fruit, White Cheddar Rice Cake, Snack Bar, a couple of Cookies and Waters.

Other things that I enjoy for lunch are:

Peanut Butter smeared into Celery stalks
An Apple cut up & dipped into Peanut Butter
Salmon or Sardines mixed into Salsa with a few Cheez Its or Cheese Puffs added just before eating. Omit the Fish if you don't like it but don't forget to include some other protein source in your meal. Salsa is an excellent value.
A hard boiled Pickled Egg
Sandwiches: Egg, Tuna, or Chicken Salad, Peanut Butter & Banana and/or Honey, Lean Lunch Meats, Leftovers like Roast Beef or Chicken, Low calorie Cheese slices, etc.
There are a nice variety of 90 calorie snack bars available. I originally tried to make my own Granola type bars but soon found that I couldn't do any better than the ones on the market. I enjoy the higher calorie Fruit and Nut bars as well.
Fresh Fruit Salad
Cole Slaw
Chocolate Chunk or Caramel Corn Rice cake with an apple! Use your imagination!

A well stocked fridge.

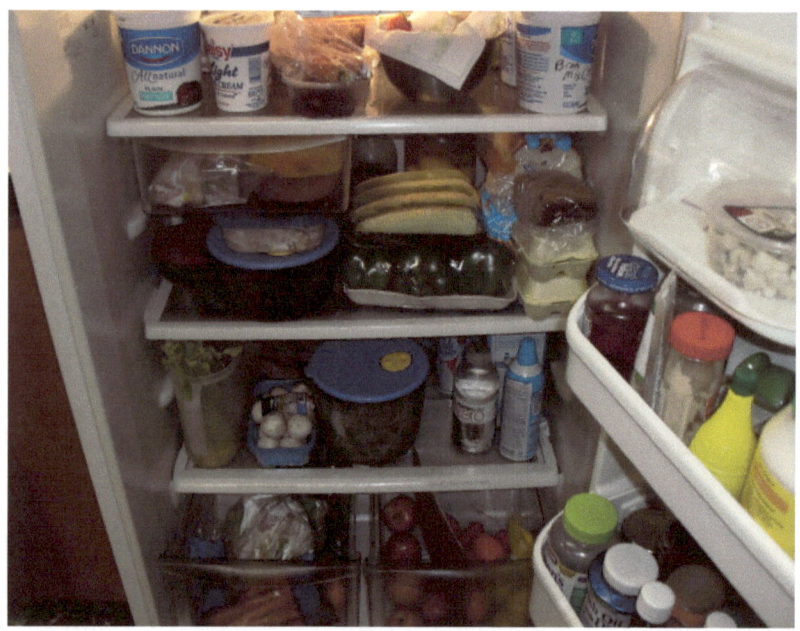

We eat a green Salad 4-5 nights per week. You can make it a Taco salad by adding a small amount of Seasoned Beef, some Fat Free Shredded Cheese, &, a few crumbled Tortilla Chips topped with Salsa, Taco Sauce, & Light Sour Cream instead of dressing. We also enjoy adding some Chicken on occasion & make the Salad the entree. I particularly enjoy Buffalo Chicken or Tarragon Chicken Salad. Delicious!

Blackened Salmon

530 Calories

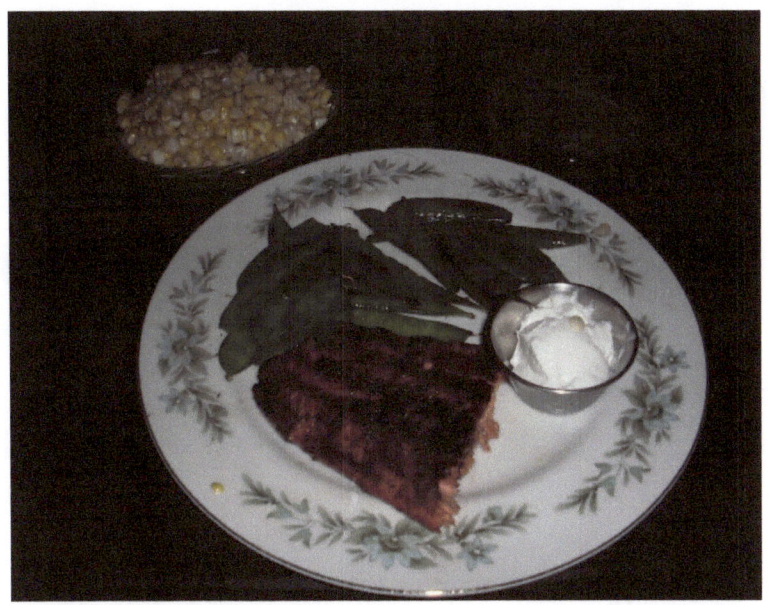

Salmon (150), Sour Cream (40), Snow & Snap Peas (40),
Corn with butter sprinkles (200), Broccoli (100)

Heat cast iron pan on the grill to very hot & then sear Fish
sprayed with Oil & seasoned with blackening seasoning.
Time depends on thickness. Fish is usually 3-5 minutes per
side. Try this with Beef. Yum!

Salad & Shrimp

300 Calories

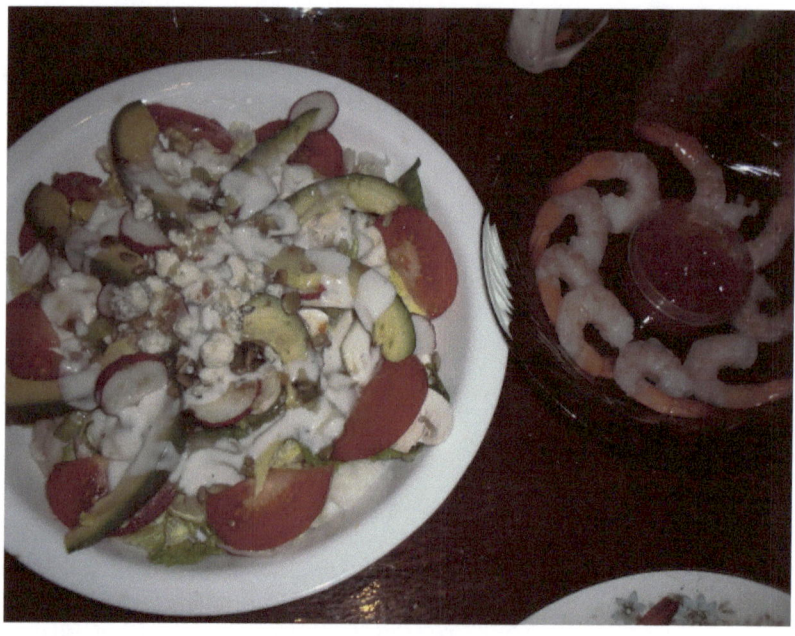

Lettuces and/or Spinach, Celery, Cucumbers, Tomatoes, Mushrooms, Radishes, Avocado, Pumpkin & Sunflower Seeds, Crumbly Bleu Cheese, & about 4T of low calorie Dressings.
Shrimp is a wonderfully inexpensive dish! 1 large Shrimp is 7 calories. These are about 6 calories each. We normally share a bag but this was for company so we stretched it to three consumers.

Example Dinners (My Favorite Meal of the Day)

Hot Dogs
497 Calories

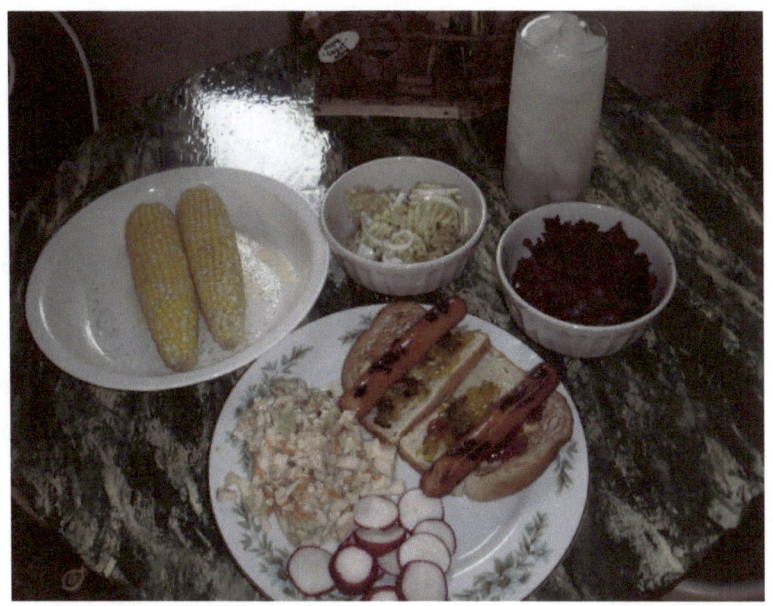

Two Fat Free Hot Dogs on low calorie Bread (180), Cole
Slaw (30), Radishes (2), Corn (200), Blue Kraut (40),
Cucumbers (45)
We often have hot dogs on Sunday night after church
because they are quick, easy, & low calorie as well as
delicious!

Foil Wrapped Seasoned Chicken Breast

800 Calories

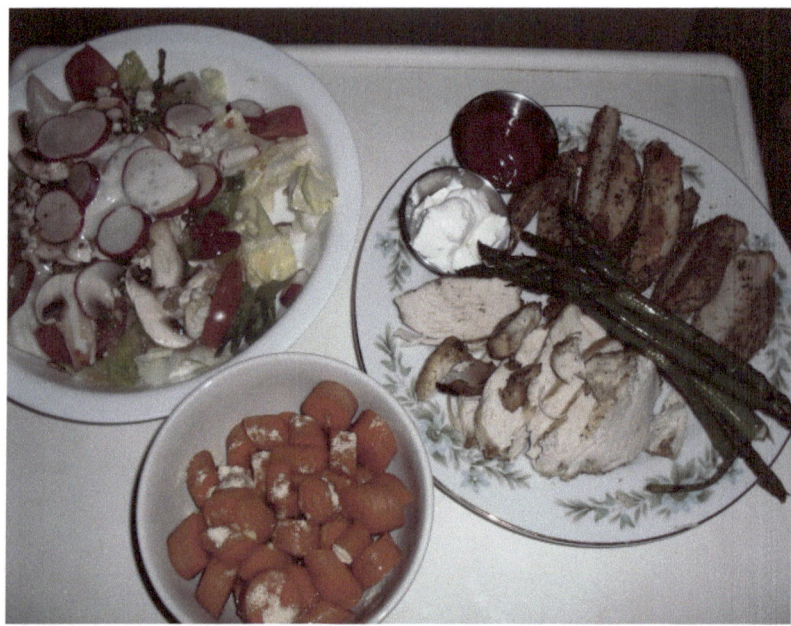

Chicken (300), Roasted Potato Wedges (160), Asparagus (30), Light Sour Cream & Ketchup (90), Carrots with butter sprinkles (70), Salad (150)

(Obviously my *husband's portions*)

Patty Melts

635 Calories

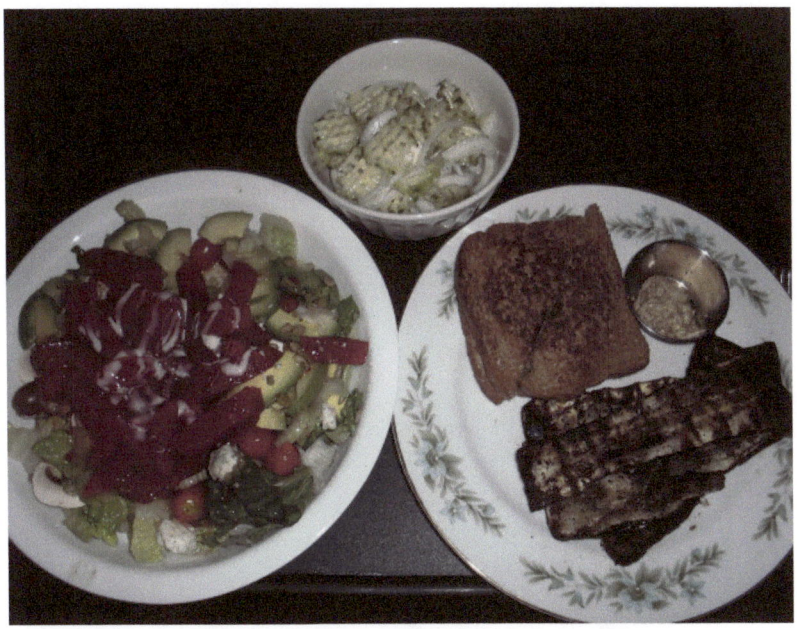

Beef Patty Melt with Horseradish Mustard (270) Use butter flavored Cooking Oil spray instead of Butter to grill, Grilled Zucchini (70), Cucumbers (45), Salad with Avocado, Bleu Cheese, & Beets(250) I blacken the Beef on the grill & then put the sandwich together. The Zucchini is sprayed with 0 calorie Olive Oil spray, seasoned, & grilled on high for 10-15 minutes.

BLT's

690 Calories

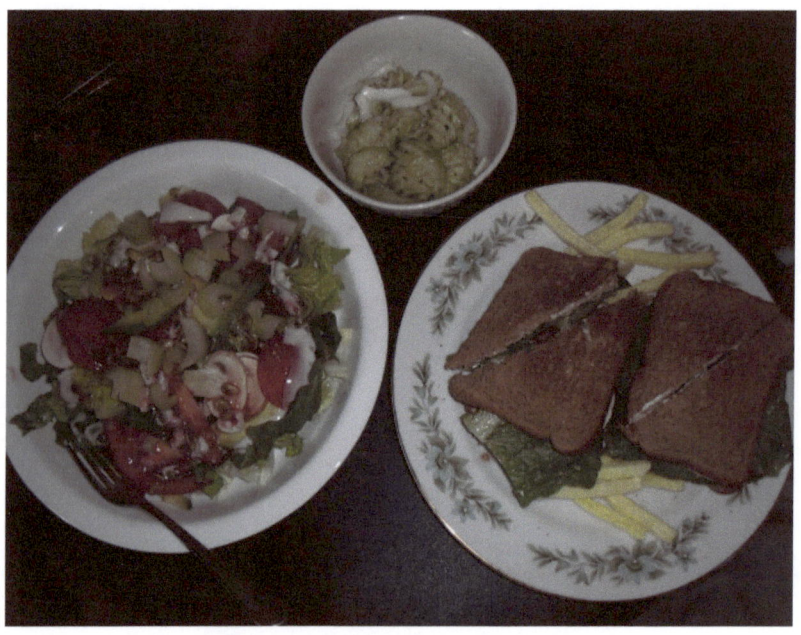

2 BLT's (360), Cucumbers (40), Potato Straws (40) Salad
with Avocado, Bleu Cheese & Seeds (250)

Sautéed Fish

595 Calories

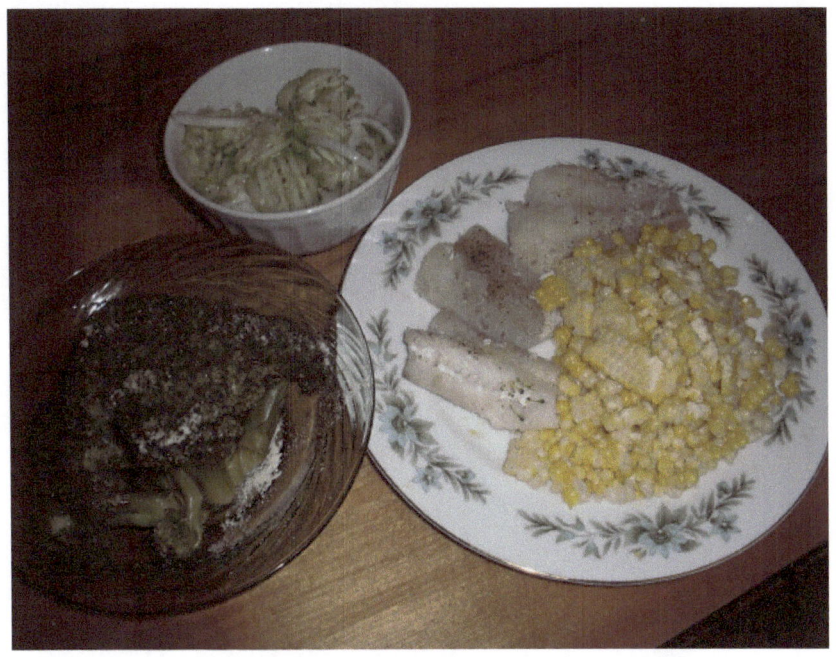

Gently Sautéed Fish (250), Corn (200), Broccoli (100),
Cucumbers (45)

Meatloaf

700 Calories

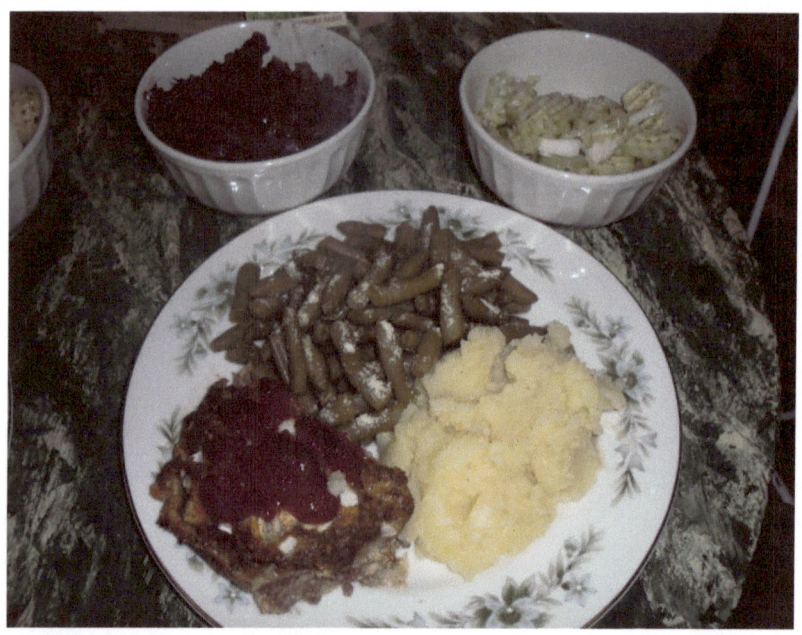

Meatloaf (350), Mashed Potatoes (200), Green Beans (70),
Blue Kraut (40), Cucumbers (40)

Pot Roast

590 Calories

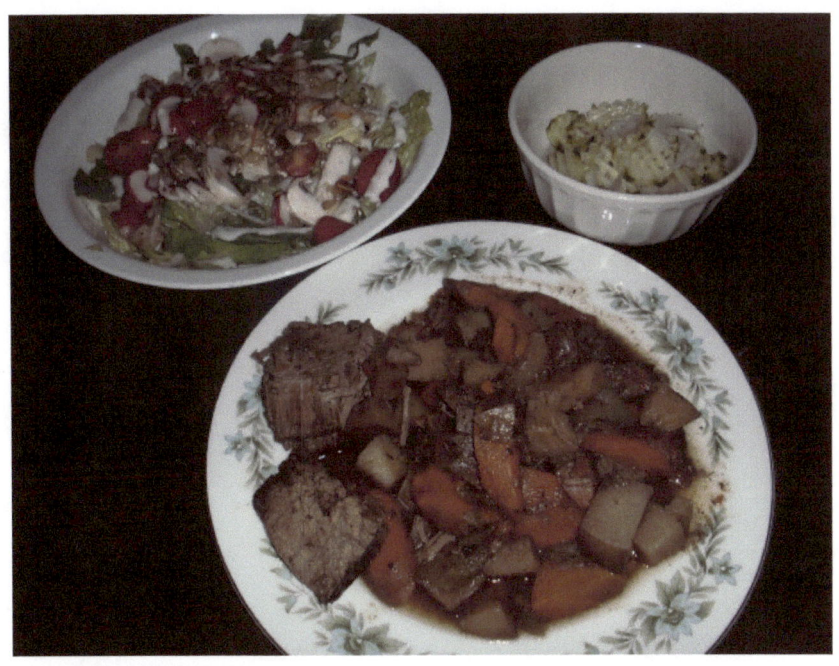

Beef Pot Roast cooked in a crockpot (200), A-1 sauce (5), Potatoes, Onions, & Carrots (175), Salad (175), Cucumbers (35)

Seasoned Chicken Salad

600 Calories

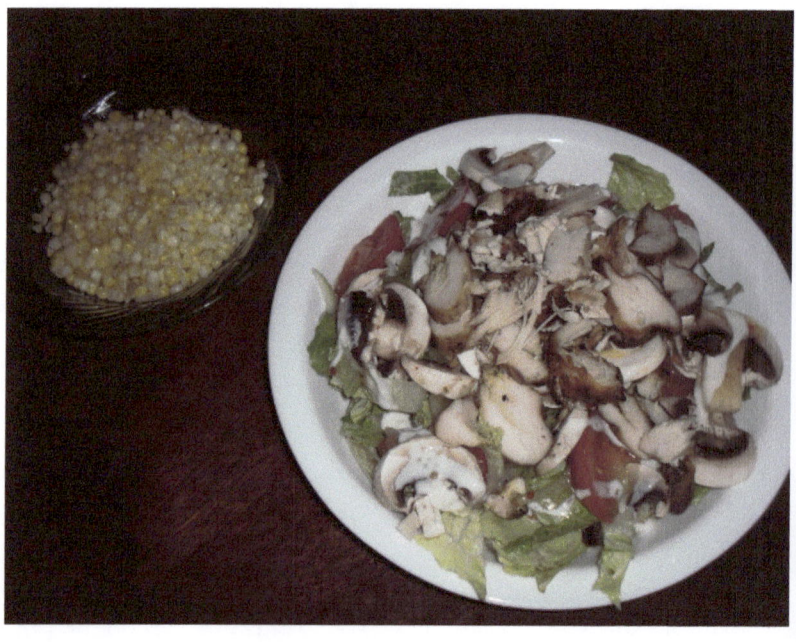

Salad with Chicken (400), 2 pieces of Corn cut off the cob with butter flavored granules (200)

Pork Chops

400 Calories

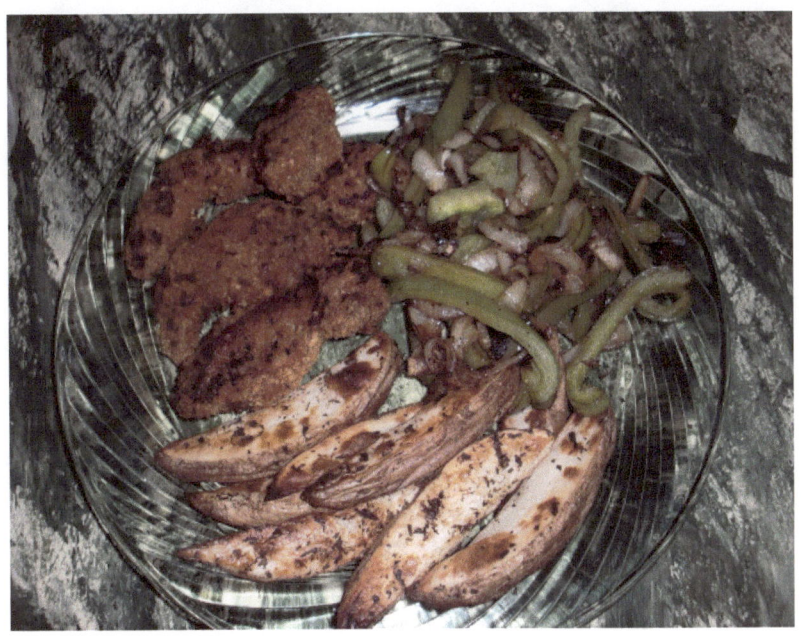

Pork Chop with all of the fat cut off & seasoned with Dijon mustard & then Shake n' Bake (230), Wedged Potatoes with cooking spray & seasonings baked near 400 til browned (150), sautéed green peppers & onions (20)

Spinach Lasagna

590 Calories

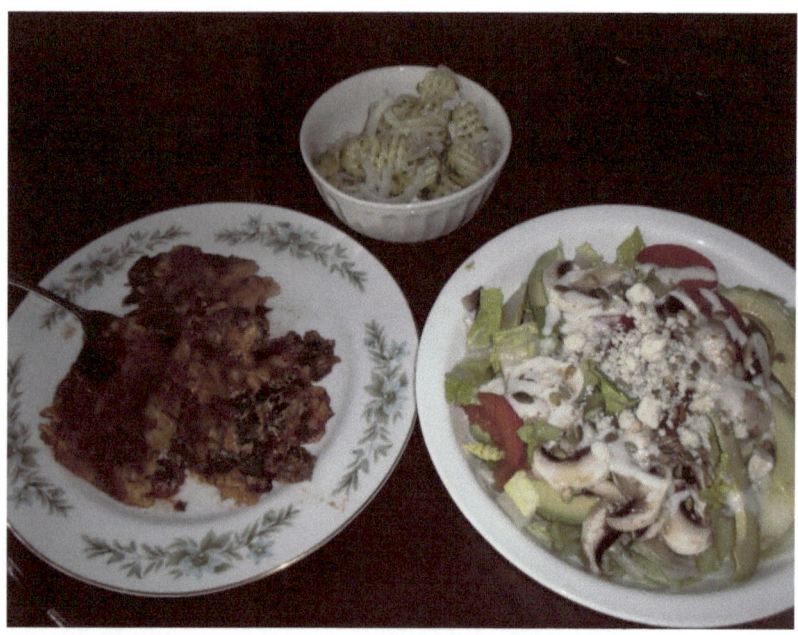

Lasagna made with Spinach instead of meat & with low fat
Cheeses (300), Cucumbers (40), Salad with the works (250)

Spaghetti Squash

565 Calories

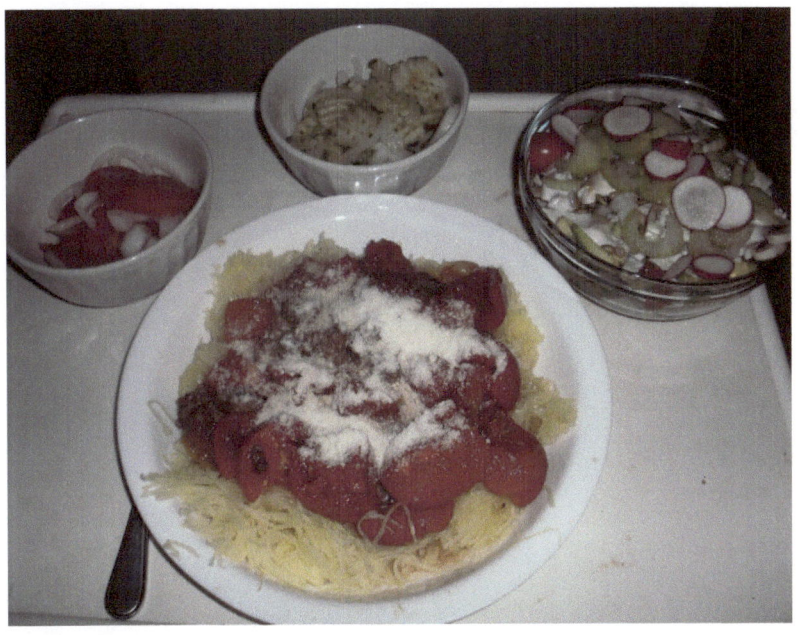

Squash & Sauce (350) Salad (125) Cucumbers (40)
Tomatoes & Onions (50)
To prepare Squash: Cut it in half, de-seed it, & then place it
upside down on a baking sheet. Bake @ 350 degrees until
tender. 30-45 minutes. Allow to cool some & then remove
Squash with a fork & then a spoon. It comes out in shreds
like spaghetti!

Taco Salad Anyone?

(A meal in itself. That's a 9x13 casserole dish.)

600 Calories

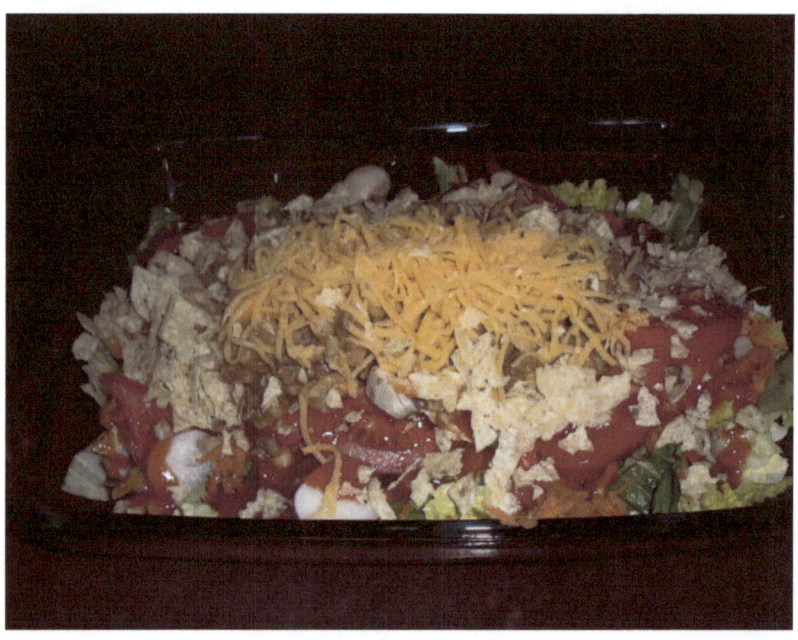

Delicious & Nutritious!

How about

Homemade Pizza Pie?

250 Calories per 1/16th of pie

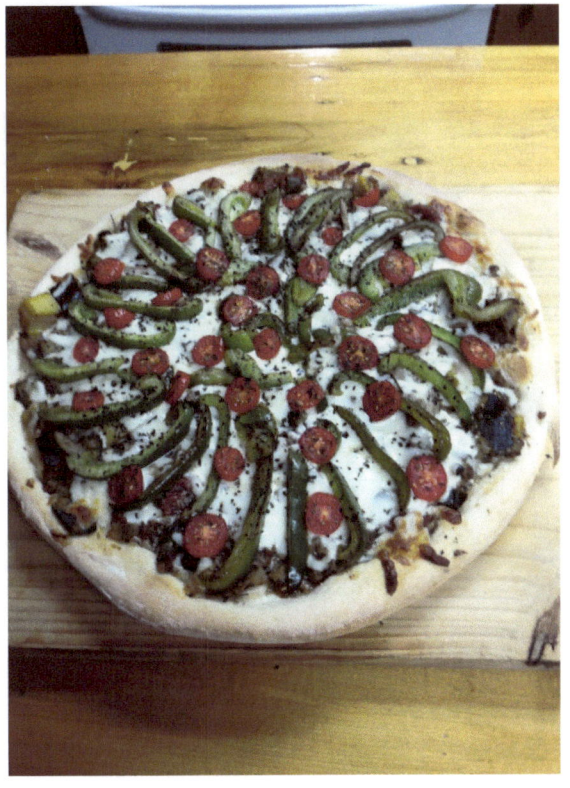

The Crust is the culprit but worth every bite!

Typical Desserts   (OK! **_THIS_** IS MY FAVORITE MEAL!)

His Banana Split and her Whipped Cream Madness

500 and 380 Calories

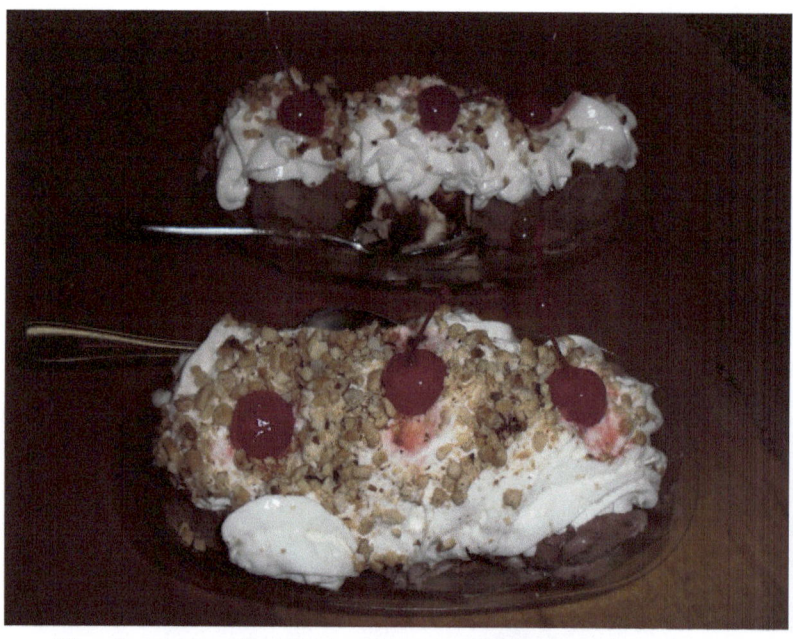

His: 3 scoops of Light Ice Cream (250) Chocolate &
Caramel Sauces (80), Fat Free Whipped Cream (20), Nuts
(20), Banana (100), Cherries (30)
Hers: 3 scoops Light Ice Cream (250), Whipped Cream
(60), Nuts (40), Cherries (30)

Sugar Free Peach Jell-O with Mangos

90 Calories

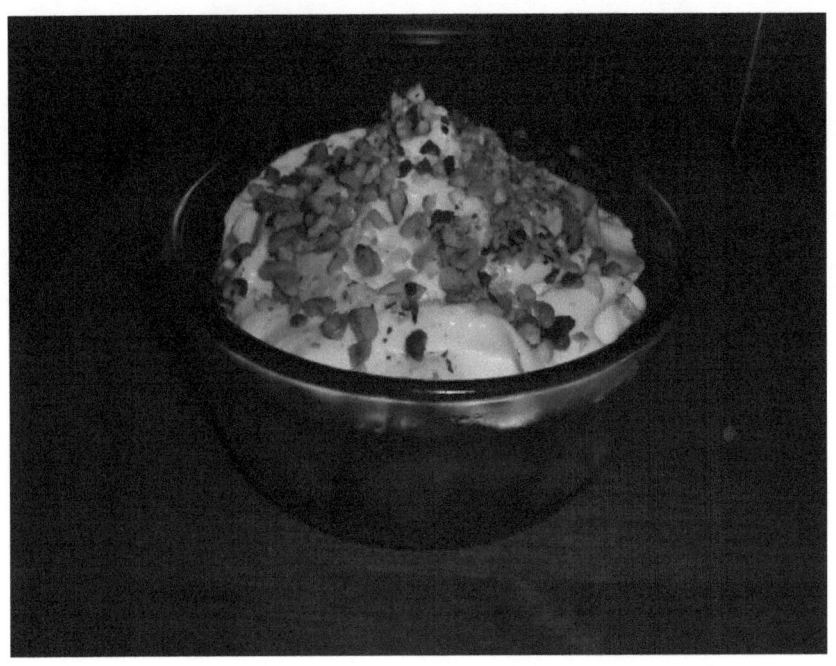

Jell-O (20), Mango (20), Whipped Cream (15), Nuts (35)

Deluxe Chocolate Ice Cream Cone

340 Calories

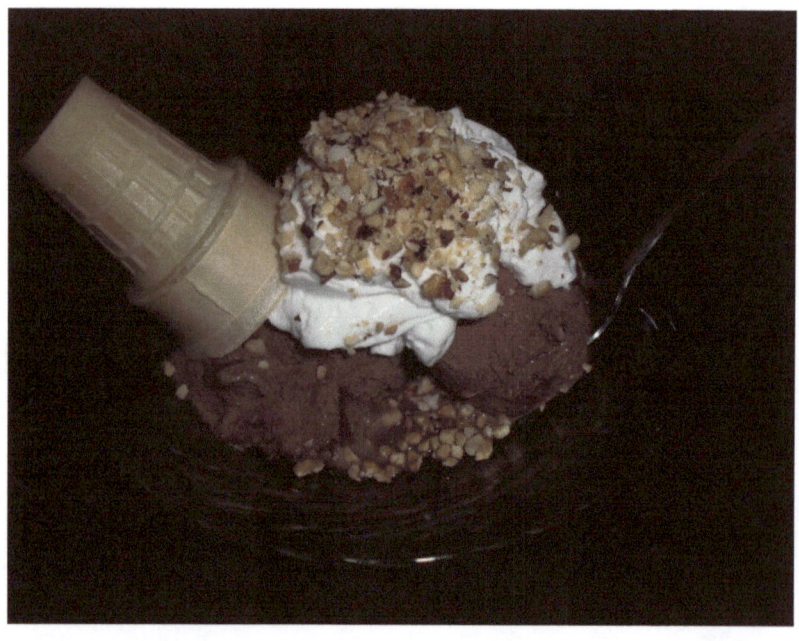

Light Ice Cream (250), Fat Free Whipped Cream (20), Nut
Topping (50), Cone (20)

Glazed Strawberries

100 Calories

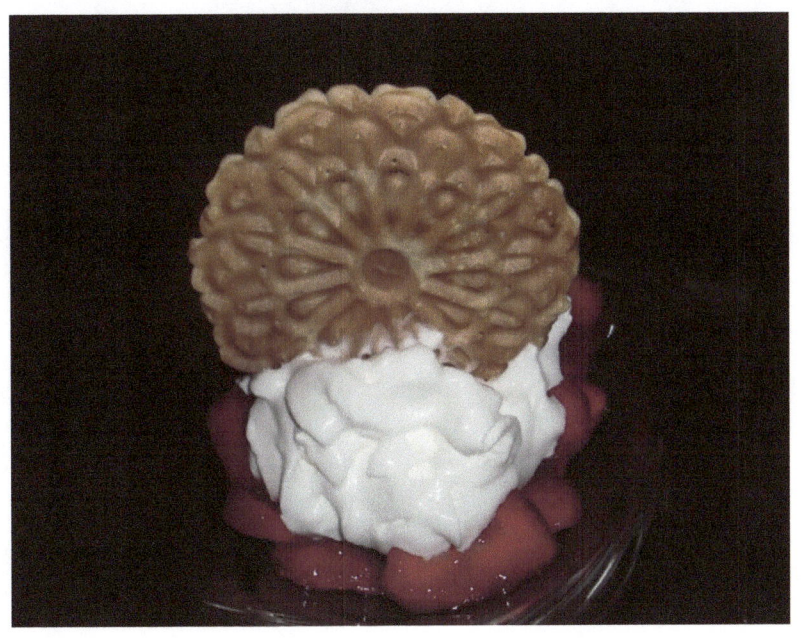

Sugar Free Strawberry Glaze mixed into Strawberries (50), Whipped Cream (25) & a Pizelle (25)

Ice Cream Float

130 Calories

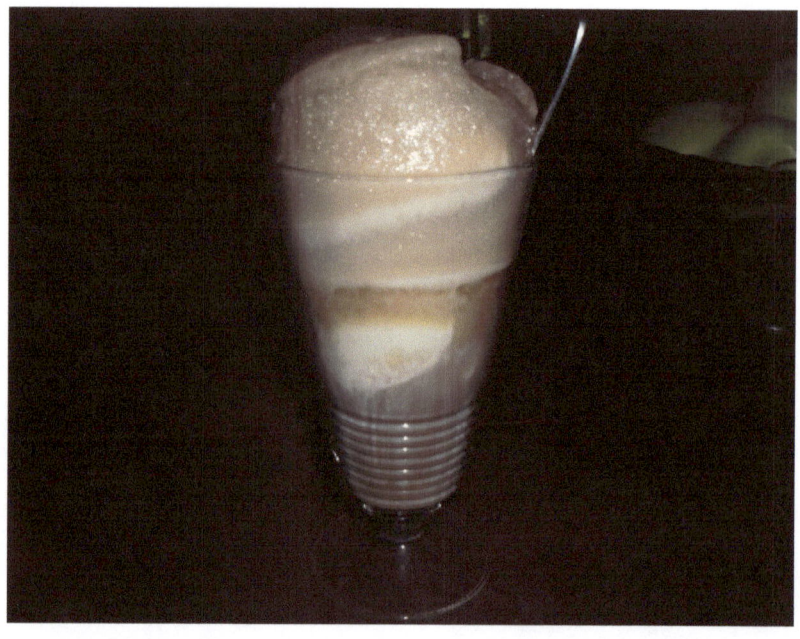

You only count the ice cream so it's easy to figure. Great filler upper!

There are many possibilities for low calorie desserts.

Some examples include:

A boxed Cake mix baked with just 12 oz. of diet soda instead of oil, eggs, & water & with Fat Free Whipped Topping or Sugar Free Pudding as frosting. Try different soda & Cake combinations

Sugar Free Puddings. Make a Mousse by blending with Fat Free Whipped Topping

Pies made in ramekins with no Crust or with Crust on top only

Apple or Cherry Crisps using splenda

Baked Apples & Cinnamon

Fresh Fruit Salads

Use your imagination & create your own Masterpieces of enjoyment!

Some Final Points

If I were going to summarize my approach I'd say it's all about education & modification.

Once I educated myself on the calorie cost of foods I was able to modify recipes to reduce the cost. I substitute & modify at will to create delicious meals.

One such substitution is Macaroni & Cheese. My husband makes the best I've ever had but it is excessively high in calories. I made it with Spaghetti Squash instead of the Macaroni! He likes it better! I can actually use less Cheese because the Squash doesn't mask the Cheese flavor as much as the Macaroni did & the Squash has a fraction of the calories in Pasta.

For Spaghetti Squash & Cheese follow a Macaroni & Cheese recipe. Substitute the Macaroni with baked Spaghetti Squash & reduce the Cheese by half or so.
See page 41 for Spaghetti Squash preparation.
I mix the Squash with Cheddar Cheese, Milk, & Onions. Fill the baking dish half way, add a layer of thin Muenster Cheese, & then fill with the rest of the Squash mixture. Bake for 45 minutes covered @ 350 degrees. Then top with 2 slices of cubed Bread & uncover. Bake for 15 minutes more. Amazing!

I love looking at recipe magazines. The pictures inspire me to create new menu items. I rarely follow the recipe exactly.

I recently learned that my cholesterol is a bit high & I'm now modifying my diet to facilitate the increase of my HDL & reduction of my LDL levels. That's another subject & it is an easy adjustment. I found all of the information that I needed online. I am increasing my ingestion of Beans, Oatmeal, Nuts, etc.

The weight management techniques that I've described herein promote a healthy lifestyle. Everyone is different & you should adjust your regimen accordingly if you have any special concerns.

I hope that this little book is helpful to you. I was motivated to write it because I wanted to share the success that we've achieved. It feels so good to be carrying around the appropriate amount of weight. My prayer is that you'll enjoy the same success. Enjoy the process & the FOOD!

YOU CAN DO THIS!

www.ingramcontent.com/pod-product-compliance
Lightning Source LLC
Chambersburg PA
CBHW050829290526
45792CB00001B/315